Anti Inflammatory Healthy Diet Cookbook

Quick and Easy Anti-Inflammatory Recipes breakfast, lunch, dinner, Anti-Inflammatory Diet Recipes

By

Gary P. Torres

Under no circumstances will any legal responsibility or blame be held against the publisher for any reparation, damages, or monetary loss due to the information herein, either directly or indirectly.

Respective authors own all copyrights not held by the publisher.

The information herein is offered for informational purposes solely, and is universal as so. The presentation of the information is without contract or any type of guarantee assurance.

The trademarks that are used are without any consent, and the publication of the trademark is without permission or backing by the trademark owner. All trademarks and brands within this book are for clarifying purposes only and are the owned by the owners themselves, not affiliated with this document.

Table of contents

Introduction

This book contains proven steps and strategies on how to serve breakfast, lunch and dinner meals for people who undergo an anti-inflammatory diet. An anti- inflammatory diet is recommenced for people who suffer from serious diseases such as rheumatoid arthritis.

It contains a list of six breakfast recipes, six lunch recipes and six dinner recipes. Each recipe shows the needed ingredients, procedures and health information such as calorie count, fat content, cholesterol amount and sodium content. For health purposes, it's recommended to follow the recipe before replacing core ingredients with your preferred ones.

Chapter 1: About the Anti Inflammatory Diet

Chronic inflammation affecting the human body can cause serious diseases such as Alzheimer's, cancer, rheumatoid arthritis and heart diseases. Normally, inflammation is the body's reaction to infection or injury. Signs of inflammation are swelling, redness and pain. However, when it lasts longer or when it appears without any apparent reason, it is a sign that the body is taking damage. Lifestyle habits such as smoking, stressful work, lack of exercise and unhealthy meals can trigger chronic inflammation.

For a patient to fight inflammation and to prevent it from getting serious, he/she has to undergo an anti-inflammatory diet. Aside from helping with weight loss, the diet plan can also help prevent diseases. It aids in keeping a patient's health in balance.

1.1 Contents of an anti-inflammatory diet

An anti-inflammatory diet should contain a recommended daily intake of 2,000 – 3,000 calories, 67 grams of fat and 2,300 mg of sodium. Fifty percent (50%) of those calories should come from carbohydrates, twenty percent (20%) should come from protein and the remaining thirty percent (30%) should come from fat. You can get carbohydrate-rich foods from eating whole-wheat grains, sweet potatoes, squash, bulgur wheat, beans and brown rice.

On the other hand, your intake of fat should come from most types of fish and any foods cooked in extra-virgin olive oil or organic canola oil. You can get protein from soybeans and other whole-soy products.

This diet prohibits fast food or processed food in any part of the meal. This also means a restriction on pork, beef, butter, cream and margarine. The anti- inflammatory diet should also contain less processed sugar for diabetics and low cholesterol (though Omega-3, which is found in a variety of fish, is a good cholesterol) for people with heart problems.

1.2 Benefits of an anti-inflammatory diet

One of the benefits of an anti-inflammatory diet is that it uses fresh foods with phytonutrients that prevent degenerative ailments from occurring. The diet plan also produces cardiovascular benefits; thanks to the inclusion of the Omega-3 fatty acids. These fatty acids aid in preventing complications in the heart and reducing the levels of "bad" cholesterol and blood pressure.

Another benefit of the anti-inflammatory diet is that it is diabetic friendly. As this diet restricts processed sugar and sugar-loaded meals and snacks, it works perfectly for patients who are suffering diabetes. While the diet does not substantially reduce weight, it decreases a patient's likelihood of suffering from obesity. This is due to the inclusion of natural fruits and vegetables, and the restriction of meat and other processed foods.

Chapter 2: Breakfast Recipes

Recipe # 1 – Ginger Apple Muffins

Ingredients:

All-purpose flour (2 cups)

Sugar or sugar-free sweeteners (2/3 cup) Baking powder (1 tbsp.)

Salt (1/2 tsp.)

Ground cinnamon (1 tsp.) Ground ginger (1 tsp.)

Unsweetened almond milk (3/4 cup) - To make almond milk, you'll need to soak almonds in water for 1 – 2 days, drain and rinse them, then grind them with fresh water in a blender.

Shredded apple (1 cup) Mashed ripe banana (1/2 cup) Apple cider vinegar (1 tbsp.)

Procedure:

Pre-heat the oven to 400'F.

Lightly grease the molds in a muffin pan, or use parchment paper to line up the molds.

Whisk together the flour, sugar, baking powder, salt, cinnamon and ginger in a mixing bowl until you form a smooth batter without any lumps.

In another mixing bowl, mix the almond milk, shredded apples, mashed banana and apple cider vinegar until the mixture is fully combined. Add the flour mixture and stir until the batter incorporates the milk mixture.

Fill the batter into the muffin molds, until the molds are 2/3 full.

Bake the muffins into the oven at 400'F for 15 – 20 minutes. When you insert a toothpick into a muffin and it comes clean, they are ready.

The ginger apple muffins yield 12 servings, with each muffin at approximately

170 calories. It has 0.6 mg fat, zero cholesterol, and 234 mg sodium.

Recipe # 2 – Spinach and Mushroom Frittatas

Ingredients:

Sliced button mushrooms (1 lb.) Chopped large onion (1 pc.)
Chopped garlic (1 tbsp.) Spinach (1 lb.)

Water (1/4 cup) Egg whites (6 pcs.) Eggs (4 pcs.)

Firm tofu (6 oz.)

Ground turmeric (1/2 tsp.) Kosher salt (1/2 tsp.)

Cracked or powdered black pepper (1/2 tsp.)

Procedure:

Pre-heat the oven to 350'F.

In a non-stick skillet or sauté pan, sauté the button mushrooms over medium to high heat. Add chopped onions and keep sautéing for 3 minutes or until the onions are tender.

Add water. Then add spinach to the skillet or pan and cook for 2 minutes with the lid on, or until the spinach wilts. Cook again until all the water is dispersed. Set aside.

Puree, eggs, turmeric, salt, pepper, tofu and egg whites in a blender at medium or high speed until the mixture is smooth.

Gently pour the egg mixture into the spinach.

Bake the sauté pan into the oven for 25 – 30 minutes at 350'F. Once it's done, take the pan out, invert the frittata onto a plate and leave it for 10 minutes. Once it's done, cut the frittata into wedges and they're ready to be served.

The frittatas yield 6 – 8 servings. Each serving has 130 g fat, 123mg cholesterol and 362mg sodium.

Recipe # 3 – Gluten-Free Strawberry Crepes

Ingredients:

Sliced strawberries (6 cups) Sugar or honey (2 tbsp.) Large eggs (4 pcs.)

Unsweetened almond milk (1 cup) Olive oil (2 tbsp.)

Vanilla extract (1 tsp.) Light brown sugar (1 tsp.) Salt (1 tsp.)

Gluten-free flour baking mix (3/4 cup)

Procedures:

Mix strawberries and sugar until the strawberries are coated. Let it stand for 30 minutes at room temperature.

Put the eggs, almond milk, olive oil, vanilla extract, brown sugar and salt into a mixing bowl, then whisk it all together until all the ingredients are combined.

Add the gluten-free four and mix it until the batter is smooth and creamy.

Heat a non-stick skillet or crepe pan in a stove or oven on medium heat. Add ¼ cup of batter into the skillet and coat it evenly. Cook it for around 45 seconds or until the crepe starts to turn brown.

Flip the crepe over and cook the other side for 10 seconds then transfer it to a serving plate.

Take out ½ cup of the sugared strawberries with a spoon then put it on top of the crepe. Carefully fold the crepe as you cover the strawberries, in order to form a half-circle.

Drizzle the crepe with any syrup or juice then serve.

You will need to serve two strawberry crepes to make one serving. Each serving has 220 calories, 9.7g fat, 123 mg cholesterol and 130 mg sodium.

Recipe # 4 – Cherry Quinoa Porridge

Ingredients:

Water (1 cup)

Dry quinoa (1/2 cup)

Dried unsweetened cherries (1/2 cup) Vanilla extract (1/2 tsp.)

Ground cinnamon (1/4 tsp.) Honey (1 tsp.)

Procedures:

1.   Stir together water, quinoa, cherries, vanilla extract and cinnamon in a medium-sized saucepan. Bring it to a boil over medium or high heat.

2.   Simmer with the lid covering the saucepan for 15 minutes. The quinoa is ready when all the water has been absorbed and the porridge is tender.

3.   Drizzle with honey then serve.

The quinoa porridge makes two servings. Each serving contains 314 calories, 2.8g fat, zero cholesterol and 9 mg sodium.

Recipe # 5 – Raspberry Green Tea Smoothie

Ingredients:

Chilled green tea (1 ½ cups)

Frozen unsweetened raspberries (2 cups) Banana (1 pc.)

Honey (1 tbsp.)

Protein powder (1/4 cup)

Procedure:

1.   Add all the ingredients into a blender.

2. Puree the ingredients until the mixture is very smooth and creamy.

3. Pour the puree into a tall glass and serve.

Each smoothie is equal to two cups. One smoothie has 180 calories, 1 g fat, zero cholesterol and 89 mg sodium.

Recipe # 6 – Buckwheat and Quinoa Granola

Ingredients:

Honey (3 tbsp.)

Liquid coconut oil (3 tbsp.) Vanilla extract (1 tsp.) Ground cinnamon (1/4 tsp.) Ground ginger (1/4 tsp.) Buckwheat oats (1 cup) Cooked quinoa (1 cup) Regular oats (1/2 cup)

Dried unsweetened cranberries (1/2 cup)

Procedures:

1. Line a baking sheet with parchment paper or silicon baking mat, or lightly grease a sheet with olive oil. Preheat the oven to 325'F.

2. Stir together coconut oil, vanilla extract, honey, ginger and cinnamon into a small mixing bowl.

3. In a separate large mixing bowl, mix the buckwheat, quinoa and oats together.

4. Add the honey mixture and stir thoroughly until all the ingredients are fully combined.

5. Spread the mixture evenly in a pan and bake at 325'F for 40 – 45 minutes or until it begins to brown.

6. Remove the pan and add the cranberries. Stir it well then place the pan on a cooling rack for it to cool completely.

7. Store the granola in an airtight container.

The buckwheat and quinoa granola can yield six servings. Each ¾ cup of granola contains 327 calories, 5.5 g fat, zero cholesterol and 4 mg sodium.

Recipe # 7 – Cherry Quinoa Porridge

Serves 2; Preparation time - 2 minutes Ingredients:

Water (1 cup)

Dry quinoa (1 cup)

Dried unsweetened cherries (1 cup) Vanilla extract (1/2 tsp)

Ground cinnamon (¼ tsp) Honey (¼ tsp), optional

Procedures:

1.   Get a medium-sized saucepan and stir all the ingredients (except honey) together. Over medium-high heat, bring everything to a boil.

2.   Lower the heat, cover the saucepan and simmer. Wait for 15 minutes or until the water is completely absorbed and the quinoa is all tender.

3.   If desired, drizzle with some honey before serving.

Recipe # 8 – Gingerbread Oatmeal

Serves 1; Preparation time – 10 minutes

Ingredients:

Water (1 cup)

Old-fashioned oats (½ cup)

Dried, unsweetened cranberries or cherries (¼ cup) Ground ginger (1 tsp)

Ground cinnamon (½ teaspoon) Ground nutmeg (¼ teaspoon)
Flaxseeds (1 tablespoon)

Molasses (1 tablespoon)

Procedures:

1.	Mix the water, oats, cranberries or cherries, ginger, cinnamon, and nutmeg in a small-sized saucepan and heat over medium high settings. Bring the mixture into a boil, then reduce the heat. Simmer for 5 minutes or until such time that the water has been almost completely absorbed.

2.	Put the flaxseeds, then cover the saucepan. Let the mixture stand for another 5 minutes.

3.	Drizzle the dish with some molasses before serving.

Recipe # 9 – Spanish Frittata

Serves 4 to 6

Ingredients (for the frittata):

Large organic eggs (1 dozen) Coconut milk (½ cup)

Sea salt (½ tsp, or more to taste)

Extra-virgin olive oil or coconut oil (2 tbsp) Small, finely chopped red onion (1 pc)

Sautéed mushrooms or vegetable of your choice (½ cup) Spinach or arugula (1 cup)

Procedures:

1.   Pre-heat the oven set at a temperature of 375°F.

2.   Whisk the coconut milk and eggs together as you sprinkle two pinches of salt; then set aside.

3.   Get a pan and heat coconut oil at medium-high setting. Sauté onions for about 3 minutes or until translucent. Add the mushrooms or vegetables of your choice and sauté until they soften. Put the spinach in and fold into the vegetable mixture just until they wilt. Remove the veggies from the pan and set aside.

4.   Adjust the heat to low setting, while adding just a bit more coconut oil, if necessary. With the same skillet, place the eggs while shaking to evenly distribute the mixture. Set the heat to medium-low then cook for about 5 more minutes. Use a spatula to gather the eggs at the edges and mix them with the rest of the ingredients at the center. Do this until there are no more runny edges. Arrange the veggie mix evenly over the top.

5.   Move the dish to the oven and resume cooking for 5 more minutes or until it is set and browned slightly. Turn off the heat and take the dish out of the oven; be wary of the hot handle as you do this so it is best to wear oven mitts first. Finish everything off by sliding the slightly cooked frittata onto a big serving plate. Place a plate on top of the pan. Hold together the pan and the plate then invert them in a way that the frittata falls on the plate. Slide it back to the pan so that the slightly cooked side is on top. Put the dish back into the oven and cook for another 3 or 4 minutes. Serve with a simple siding of salad with citrus vinaigrette.

Recipe # 10 – Orange Apple Breakfast Shake

Serves 1; Preparation time – 10 minutes

Ingredients

Almonds (2 tbsp.) Apple slices (1/2 cup)

Orange sections (1/2 cup) 2% milk (1 cup)

Zone Protein Powder (14g)

Procedures:

1.   Place all ingredients together in the blender. Mix until everything is well- incorporated and smooth.

2.   Pour the contents of the blender into a tall glass.

3.   Serve and enjoy!

Recipe # 11 – Chocolate Cherry Shake

Serves 1

Ingredients:

Unprocessed, unsweetened cocoa powder (1 tbsp.) Frozen dark cherries, pitted (½ cup)

Coconut, almond or flax milk (1 cup)

Pure vanilla extract; a few drops of liquid stevia preferably Sweet Leaf Vanilla Crème (½ tsp)

Ice cubes, if desired

Procedures:

1.   Mix all the ingredients in a blender. Process until everything is smooth.

2.   Pour in a tall glass.

3.   Serve and enjoy!

Recipe # 12 – Oatmeal Spiced w/ Apple Pie

Serves 4; Preparation time – 45 minutes

Ingredients:

Water (3 cups)

Steel Cut Oats (3/4 cup)

Pumpkin Spice - Pumpkin Pie Spice (2 tsp) Zone Protein Powder (70 grams) Applesauce (1 cup)

Stevia Extract (1 tsp, to taste)

16 Pecans or walnuts (16 pcs – halves)

Procedures:

1.   Boil the water before stirring in the pumpkin pie spice and steel-cut oats. Cook for about 5 minutes then reduce the heat. Simmer for half an hour. Let the dish col off before stirring in the protein powder. (This can be prepared the previous evening, refrigerate, and then just heat in the microwave oven the following morning.) Add the rest of the ingredients once you are about to eat.

2.   If prepared the previous night, take the dish out of the refrigerator and pour into 4 individual bowls. Distribute the rest of the ingredients among the 4 bowls and warm up in the microwave oven for 2 ½ minutes under high temperature setting. Stir while halfway through.

Recipe # 13 – Eggs and Apple Pork w/ Strawberries

Serves 1

Ingredients:

Olive oil (1 1/2 tsps - divided)

Boneless center-cut loin pork chops (2 oz) Salt & pepper, to taste

Small apple, sliced (1 pc) Cinnamon (1/4 tsp)

Egg whites (1/2 cup) Strawberries, sliced (1 cup)

Procedures:

1. Heat half a teaspoon of olive oil in a large skillet under medium-high. Place the salt & pepper-seasoned pork, and the cinnamon-seasoned apple slices on opposite sides of the skillet.

2. Cook until the pork is no longer pinkish and the apple slices are just a bit soft.

2. Remove the pork and apple slices from the skillet, and set aside. Keep warm.

3. Heat the remaining 1 tsp of olive oil and scramble the egg whites.

4. Garnish the dish with some sliced strawberries on the side.

5. Serve and enjoy!

Recipe # 14 – Eggs and Fruit Salad

Serves 1; Preparation time – 20 minutes

Ingredients:

Strawberries, sliced (1/2 cup)

Mandarin orange sections, unsweetened or fresh (1/2 cup) Blueberries (1/2 cup)

Egg whites (6 hardboiled eggs, discard yolks) Avocado (1/2 cup)

Salsa (3 tbsp.)

Procedures:

1.   Prepare the fruit salad in a medium-sized bowl. Slice strawberries, and then gently stir blueberries and mandarin sections in.

2.   Boil the eggs for about 10 minutes, then allow to cool. Halve the eggs and remove the yolks.

3.   Dice the hardboiled egg whites and avocado; mix in a separate bowl. Stir the salsa in.

4.   Put some fruit salad sidings, and serve.

Recipe # 15 – Ham & Onion Frittata w/ Fruit Salad

Serves 4; Preparation time – 30 minutes

Ingredients:

Cooking spray (olive oil) Onion, chopped (1 pc)

Canadian bacon, cut in bite sized pieces (4 oz) Egg whites (2 cups)

Olive oil (1 tbsp.) 1% milk (1/4 cup)

Dried dill (1 tbsp or 3 tbsp if fresh) Salt and pepper, to taste

Mozzarella cheese, shredded (3/4 cup) Parmesan cheese, grated (1/4 cup) Blueberries (1 cup, divided)

Freshly squeezed lemon juice (3 tbsp) Vanilla 1 1/2 tsps

Agave nectar (1 ½ tbsp.) Peach, sliced (1 pc) Pear, sliced (1pc)

Strawberries, sliced (1 ½ cups)

Procedures:

1.   Spray olive oil in a large ovenproof skillet. Saute the ham and onion until the onion is cooked and golden. Set them aside.

2.   Pre-heat the oven for broiling.

3.   Whisk together the egg whites, milk, olive oil, dill, and salt & pepper in a medium-sized bowl. Add the cheeses into the mix.

4.   Spread the cooled ham and onion evenly at the bottom of the skillet. Top with the egg mixture. Cook under medium heat setting until the bottom settles.

5.   Put the skillet under broiler, and then cook some more until the eggs are set and the top is golden brown. Remove the skillet from the oven and set it aside and allow to cool off.

6.   Take ¼ cup of blueberries and mix with vanilla, agave nectar, and lemon

juice in a small-sized bowl. Set the mixture aside.

7.   Mix the sliced fruits and blueberries in a large-sized bowl. Pour the sauce mixture over the fruits and mix everything up.

8.   Serve and enjoy with the frittata.

Recipe # 16 – Grapefruit Breakfast

Serves 1; Preparation time – 5 minutes

Ingredients:

Canadian bacon (2 slices) Grapefruit (1 pc)

0%-fat Greek yogurt (1/2 cup) Blueberries (1/3 cup)

Sliced almonds (3 1/2 tbsp.)

Procedures:

1.   Get the slices of Canadian bacon and cut into smaller pieces. Place in the microwave oven to warm.

2.   Cut the grapefruit into two, then slice each section into smaller pieces. Place the pieces in a bowl. Stir the Canadian bacon in.

3.   Next, get another bowl and mix the almonds and blueberries with yogurt.

4.   Combine the contents of the two bowls and mix well.

5.   Serve and enjoy!

Chapter 3: Lunch Recipes

Recipe # 1 – Roasted Chicken Wraps

Ingredients:

Low-fat or reduced-fat mayonnaise (1/2 cup) Pickle juice (2 tbsp.)

Freshly cracked black pepper (1 tsp.) Shredded red cabbage (1 ½ cups) Apple cider vinegar (1 tbsp.)

Kosher salt (1/4 tsp.) Cayenne pepper (1/4 tsp.)

Cooled deli roasted chicken (1 whole)

Wheat, whole-wheat or mixed-grain flatbreads (6 pcs.)

Procedures:

1.   Mix pickle juice, pepper and mayonnaise in a mixing bowl. Put the mixture into the refrigerator to set aside.

2.   Meanwhile, add salt, vinegar, cabbage and cayenne pepper into a separate mixing bowl. Toss the cabbage to mix it with the other ingredients.

3.   Discard skin and bones from the roasted chicken and shred the chicken into bite-sized pieces.

4.   Add the chicken into the mayonnaise mixture and combine it.

5.   Arrange the cabbage and the chicken evenly in the flatbread slices and roll it tightly.

6.   You can either eat it on its own, or heat it using a toaster oven or microwave oven.

Each chicken wrap contains 286 calories, 8.2g fat, 59mg cholesterol and 239 mg sodium.

Recipe # 2 – Lentil and Garbanzo Soup

Ingredients:

Chopped onions (2 pcs.) Chopped celery (1 cup) Diced carrots (1 cup) Grated ginger (2 tsp.) Minced garlic (1 tsp.) Garam masala (1 tsp.) Turmeric (1 tsp.) Ground cumin (1/2 tsp.)

Ground cayenne pepper (1/4 tsp.) Vegetable broth or stock (6 cups) Lentils (1 cup)

Rinsed and drained garbanzo beans (2 15-oz. cans) Undrained petite diced tomatoes (1 14.5-oz. can)

Procedures:

1.   Sauté onions in a large pot over medium to high heat for 3 – 4 minutes or until onions are tender.

2.   Add celery and carrots into the pot and keep cooking for an additional five minutes. Stir in garlic, garam masala, turmeric, cumin and cayenne pepper into the pot and keep cooking for 30 more seconds.

3.   Add the cups of broth, lentils, garbanzo beans and tomatoes into the pot, then keep stirring the ingredients until all of them are combined. Cook the broth for 90 minutes or until the lentils are tender.

4.   For a creamier and thicker soup, you can take out half of the broth, puree it with a food processor, then put it back into the pot and stir.

The broth makes up eight servings, and each serving is 1 ½ cup. Each serving has 253 calories, 3.7 g fat, 5 mg cholesterol, and 604 mg sodium.

Recipe # 3 – Roasted Sweet Potato Soup

Ingredients:

Sweet potatoes (2 ½ lbs.) Extra-virgin olive oil (1 tbsp.) Kosher salt (1/4 tsp.)

Freshly cracked pepper (1/2 tsp.) Sliced leek or onions (1 ½ cups) Minced garlic (1 tsp.)

White wine (1/2 cup) Chopped thyme leaves (1 tsp.) Vegetable broth (5 cups) Orange juice (2 cups)

Procedures:

1.   Pre-heat the oven to 400'F. Peel and cut sweet potatoes into very small pieces.

2.   Place the sweet potatoes on a baking sheet and toss them with pepper, olive oil and salt. Roast the potatoes in the oven for 45 – 50 minutes at 400'F or until the sweet potatoes are well browned. Set aside.

3.   In a large soup pot, cook the leeks or onions over medium to high heat for 8 minutes or until they are tender. Add ginger and garlic, stir and cook for one more minute. Add the white wine and bring it to a boil until the wine evaporates.

4.   When all the wine has evaporated, add the vegetable broth, thyme and sweet potatoes then bring the whole soup mixture into a boil. Turn down the heat and let it simmer for 20 minutes or until the vegetables are soft and tender.

5.   Use a blender to puree the soup in batches. Reheat each batch of soup before serving.

The sweet potato soup can yield eight servings, or 1 ½ cup per serving. Each

serving has 190 calories, 3.9 g fat, 5 mg cholesterol and 324 mg sodium.

Recipe # 4 – Kipper (Smoked Herring) Salad

Ingredients:

Low-fat or reduced-fat mayonnaise (1/2 cup) Finely chopped small onion (1 pc.)

Finely chopped celery stalk (1 pc.) Chopped parsley (1 tbsp.)

Lemon juice (1 tsp.) Minced garlic (1 clove) Salt (1/8 tsp.)

Ground black pepper (1/8 tsp.)

Drained kippers or smoked herring (1 6-oz. pc.)

Procedures:

1.   Stir together all the ingredients except kipper in a medium-sized bowl.

2.   Add flaked kippers into the mixture and gently toss them.

3.   Refrigerate once the salad is done. You can use it as a sandwich filling or as a side dish to your main course.

The kipper salad can yield four servings, with each serving containing 150 calories, 9.3 g fat, 25 mg cholesterol and 298 mg sodium.

Recipe # 5 – Quick-and-Easy Pumpkin Soup

Ingredients:

Chopped onion (1 cup)

Peeled and minced gingerroot (1 1-inch pc.) Minced garlic (1 clove)

Vegetable stock (6 cups) Pumpkin puree (4 cups) Salt (1 tsp.)

Chopped thyme (1/2 tsp.) Half-and-half milk (1/2 cup) Chopped parsley (1 tsp.)

Procedures:

1. Put garlic, ginger and onion in a large soup pot. Add ½ cup of vegetable stock and cook for 5 minutes or until onion is tender.

2. Add thyme, salt, 5 ½ cups of vegetable stock and pumpkin puree into the pot. Cook the soup for 30 minutes.

3. Puree the soup using a handheld blender until it becomes smooth.

4. Take out the soup from the stove and add half-and-half milk. Stir it well, then add chopped parsley as garnish. Serve.

This pumpkin soup yields eight servings. One serving has 120 calories, 4.0 g fat, 11 mg cholesterol and 700 mg sodium.

Recipe # 6 – Persimmon and Pear Salad

Ingredients:

Whole-grain mustard (1 tsp.) Lemon juice (2 tbsp.)

Extra virgin olive oil (3 tbsp.) Minced shallot (1 pc.) Minced garlic (1 tsp.)

Sliced ripe persimmon (1 pc.) Sliced ripe pear (1 pc.)

Toasted and chopped pecans (1/2 cup) Baby spinach (6 cups)

Procedures:

1. Whisk together shallot, garlic, mustard, lemon juice and olive oil in a salad bowl.

2.   Add persimmon, spinach, pecans and pear into the salad mixture. Toss well to coat the fruits and vegetables.

3.   Serve immediately. Store the remainder in an airtight container.

The persimmon and pear salad is good for two servings. Each serving has 386 calories, 21.6 g fat, zero cholesterol and 102 mg sodium.

Recipe # 7 - Smoked Trout Tartine

Serves 4; Preparation time – 15 minutes

Ingredients:

Freshly squeezed lemon juice (2 tbsp) Extra-virgin olive oil (1 tsp)

Dijon mustard (1 tsp) Sugar (1 pinch)

Smoked trout, flaked into small bite-size pieces (¾ pound) Capers, rinsed and drained (2 tsp)

Diced roasted red peppers (½ cup)

Cannellini (white kidney), drained and rinsed (½ can - 15-ounce) Celery, finely chopped (1 stalk)

Minced onion (2 tsp)

Chopped fresh dill (1 tsp), or dried dill ((½ tsp.)

Crusty, toasted whole-grain bread (4 large, half-inch slices) Garnish: dill sprigs

Procedures:

1.   Get a large bowl and whisk the lemon juice, olive oil, mustard, and sugar together. Then add in the rest of the ingredients, except for the bread. Toss everything to mix properly.

2.   Take a slice of bread and place it on a serving plate. Spoon some trout mixture on top. If desired, garnish it with dill sprigs.

Recipe # 8 – Tropical Quinoa Salad w/ Cashew Nuts

Serves 4

Ingredients (for the quinoa):

Dried quinoa, rinsed well (1 cup) Red onion, finely chopped (½ pc)

Apple or carrot, finely chopped (1 cup) Lime juice (from 1 lime)

Honey or agave (2 tbsp.) Extra-virgin olive oil (1 tbsp.)

Large mango, chopped (1 pc; not overly ripe) Mint, finely chopped (¼ cup)

Sea salt, just to taste (1 tsp)

Freshly ground black pepper, just to taste Ginger, finely chopped (½" pc) Avocado, chopped or thinly sliced (1 pc) Cashew nuts, coarsely chopped (1 cup)

Romaine lettuce or preferred greens, roughly chopped (3 cups)

Procedures:

1.   To cook the quinoa, put 2 cups of water in a medium-sized saucepan and bring to a boil. Add the quinoa. Cover the saucepan and simmer for around 15 to 20 minutes. Set the dish aside and let it cool, spreading it out to achieve best results.

2.   Get a large bowl and toss in the chopped apple or carrot, and red onion. Whisk the lime juice, olive oil, and honey together before tossing into the bowl. Next, add the cooked and cooled quinoa to the bowl, followed by the mango. Toss well.

3.   Add the cilantro, ginger, mint, and salt and pepper (to taste) into the mix. Garnish with chopped cashews and sliced avocado.

4.   Scoop the mixture over greens. Serve at room temperature or chilled.

Recipe # 9 – Applesauce Burger w/ Spinach Salad

Serves 1; Preparation time – 15 minutes

Ingredients:

Unsweetened applesauce, or chunk style if unavailable (1/3 cup) Old fashioned oats (3 tbsp)

Dehydrated onion flakes (2 tsp, to taste) Chili powder (1/2 tsp)

Ground chicken breast (3 oz) Dressing & Spinach Salad Olive oil (1 1/2 tsps0 Vinegar (2 tsp)

Water (2 tsp)

Sugar free All Fruit - or any preferred flavor (1 tsp) Salt & pepper, to taste

Baby spinach, stems torn off (3 cups) Red onion - roughly chopped (2 slices) Tomato, cut (1/2 pc)

Strawberries, cut into chunks or just crush a few pieces to enhance the dressing (1/2 cup)

Procedures:

1.   Pre-heat the broiler.

2.	Mix together the egg whites, oatmeal, onions. and ¼ cup applesauce. Add the chicken. Mix everything well and make a burger patty.

3.	Spray non-stick coating on broiler pan. Place the burger on the rack and broil for about 5 minutes before turning over. Broil for another 5 minutes or until the meat is no longer pinkish in color.

4.	Heat the rest of the applesauce and pour over the burger. (Experiment with the amounts of applesauce and oatmeal until your reach the desired consistency.)

5.	While the burger is still cooking, whisk together some dressing ingredients with some mashed strawberries.

6.	Get a salad bowl and mix the tomato, onion, and strawberries together. Drizzle with dressing. Serve.

Recipe # 10 – Quick Chicken Stir-Fry

Serves 1; Preparation time – 20 minutes Ingredients:

Olive oil (1 1/2 tsp) Broccoli florets (2 cups) Chopped onion (3/4 cup) Snow peas (3/4 cup) Garlic, pressed (1 clove)

Boneless chicken breast, cut to bite-size pieces (3 oz.)

Garbanzo beans, low sodium, rinsed and drained (1/4 cup)

Salsa (1/4 cup)

Procedures:

1. Pre-heat the wok under medium temperature, then heat 1 tsp of olive oil.

2. Mix the vegetables and stir fry for about 2 minutes or until defrosted and hot. Remove the veggies, put in a bowl, and set aside. Heat the rest of the oil in the wok.

3. In the hot oil, press a clove of garlic, then put the chicken in, stir fry for around 4 minutes or until done.

4. Put back the cooked veggies together with the garbanzo beans into the wok. Toss everything together for 2 more minutes. Serve with some salsa on the side.

Recipe # 11 – Asparagus Frittata w/ Fruit

Serves 4; Preparation time – 25 minutes

Ingredients:

Olive oil, divided (2 tbsp.) Onion, minced (1 1/2 cups)

Asparagus, snapped off tough ends, spears diagonally cut into 1" lengths (2 lbs) Egg, lightly beaten (1 pc)

Egg whites (2 cups) Salt & pepper, to taste

Low-fat Swiss cheese, grated (4 oz.) Mandarin orange sections (1 cup, in water) Blueberries (2 cups)

Procedures:

1.   Heat 1 ½ tbsp. of olive oil under medium high heat in a 10" ovenproof frying pan.

2.   Put the onions in and cook until soft for about 3 minutes.

3.   Toss in the asparagus; reduce heat setting to medium low. Cover and cook for another 3 minutes.

4.   Beat the egg whites after adding salt & pepper, and ½ tbsp. of oil. Pour the mix into the pan and allow to cook until the bottom is almost set, but the top is still runny. Pre-heat the oven broiler while cooking.

5.   Sprinkle some cheese over the eggs and broil for about 4 to 6 minutes or until the cheese is brown and melted.

6.   While cooking the frittata, divide the fruits evenly into 4 bowls. Take the frittata out of the oven and slide into a serving dish. Cut into wedges, then serve.

Recipe # 12 – Arlecchino Salad

Serves 1; Preparation time – 15 minutes

Ingredients:

Extra virgin olive oil (1 1/2 tsp.) Freshly squeezed lemon juice (3 tbsp.) Lemon pepper (1 tsp)

Romaine lettuce, ripped (2 cups) Strawberries, sliced (1 cup) Cucumber, sliced (1 1/2 cups, 150g) Cherry tomatoes, halved (1 cup) Mushrooms, sliced (1/2 cup) Cashew nuts, smashed (1 tsp) Chunk light tuna in water (3 oz.)

Melba toast , crushed as croutons (2 pcs)

Procedures:

1.   Whisk together the extra virgin oil, lemon pepper and lemon juice in a small-sized bowl to make the dressing.

2.   Create a salad with the rest of the ingredients (including the toasts). Mix everything in a bowl, then top with the crushed melba toast.

3.   Add the dressing before serving.

Recipe # 13 – Baked Eggs w/ Wilted Baby Spinach

Serves 2: Preparation time – 35 minutes

Ingredients:

Fresh squeezed lime juice (1 tbsp, to taste) Pear, cored (1 pc, halved)

0%-Fat Greek yogurt (1/2 cup) Vanilla extract (1 tsp) Blueberries (1/2 cup)

Cooking spray

Olive oil , divided (3 tsps) Diced shallots (1/4 cup)

Baby spinach, w/ large stems removed (1 1/2 lbs) Egg whites (1 cup)

Salt & pepper, to taste

Parmesan or Asagio cheese, shredded (2 tbsp.)

Procedures:

1.   Prepare the fruit salad first. Squeeze the lime juice into a regular-sized bowl, then add the cut pear. Stir in a way that the lime juice coats the pear. Mix vanilla with yogurt, using as much as necessary. Coat the pear with lime juice again before adding to the yogurt. Put it aside and refrigerate.

2.   Pre-heat the oven to a temperature of 4000F. Lightly spray 4 ramekins or oven-safe dishes with cooking spray. Over medium low setting, heat a large-sized skillet. Add shallots and 2 tsp of olive oil. Cook for around 2 to 3 minutes.

3.   Add the spinach and salt & pepper. Cook until the spinach is wilted or around 2 to 3 minutes.

4.   Put the cheese in, and then remove from heat. Evenly distribute the wilted spinach among the 4 oven-safe dishes, creating a well at the center of each dish.

5.   Add 1 tsp of olive oil and a dash of salt & pepper with the egg whites. Divide evenly among the dishes.

6.   Put the oven-safe dishes on 1 or 2 rimmed baking sheets. Bake for around 15 to 17 minutes or until set, or as desired.

7.   Immediately serve with the fruit salad.

Recipe # 14 – Balsamic Chicken, Tomatoes & White Bean Salad

Serves 2; Preparation time – 45 minutes including marinating time

Ingredients:

Boneless skinless chicken breast (6 oz.) Salt & pepper, to taste

Garlic, crushed (2 cloves) Whole grain mustard (1 tbsp.) Balsamic vinegar (2 tbsp.) Cooking spray, olive oil

Cannellini beans, rinsed and drained (1/2 cup) Cherry tomatoes, halved (1 pint)

Low-fat feta, crumbled (1/4 cup) Arugula leaves (6 cups)

Lemon, cut into wedges, for serving (1 pc) Extra virgin olive oil (2 tsp)

Applesauce (1 cup) Pumpkin pie spice (2 tsp)

Procedures:

1.   Season the chicken with salt & pepper. Whisk some mustard, vinegar, and garlic in a ceramic dish. Coat the chicken with the mixture. Cover and place in refrigerator for 20 minutes or more.

2.   Remove the chicken from the marinade. Warm skillet under high heat. Spray chicken lightly with oil. Cook until golden or around 1 minute for each side. Lower the heat to medium low setting.

3.   Cook the chicken for around 6 to 8 minutes on both sides, or until the chicken is cooked through.

4.   Set aside a mixture of olive oil and lemon seasoned with salt & pepper.

5.   Move the chicken to a large plate. cover and allow to sit for around 5 minutes. Mix feta, tomato, beans, dressing, and arugula in a large-sized bowl. Toss everything gently, then divide into 2 plates.

6.   Slice the chicken and garnish with salad. Scoop into plates, and season with pepper.

7.   Top with applesauce and. Serve with dessert of pumpkin pie spice.

Recipe # 15 – Chicken Barbecue Salad

Serves 1; Preparation time – 20 minutes

Ingredients:

Olive oil (2 tsp)

Boneless chicken breast, diced (3 oz.) Bell peppers, strips (1 1/2 cups) Onions, diced (1/4 cup)

Cider vinegar (1/8 tsp) Worcestershire sauce (1/8 tsp) Minced garlic (1 tsp)

Zoned Barbecue Sauce (1/2 cup) Lettuce (3 cups)

Shredded cabbage - (2 cups) Salt & pepper, to taste

Procedures:

1.   Put the chicken breast, oil, pepper, vinegar, onion, garlic and Worcestershire sauce in a saute pan. Cook until the chicken is brown and the veggies are tender, then add some Zoned barbecue sauce.

2.   Cover the pan and allow to simmer for about 5 minutes or until hot, occasionally stirring to make sure the flavors blend well.

3.   Mix shredded cabbage and lettuce together, and then put the salad- cabbage mixture on a large-sized oval plate. Scoop the veggie mixture and chicken to the middle of the plate, with the salad cabbage mixture underneath.

4.   Sprinkle with a dash of salt & pepper, and then serve quickly.

Chapter 4: Dinner Recipes

Recipe # 1 – Steamed Salmon with Lemon-Scented Zucchini

Ingredients:

Sliced onion (1 pc.) Sliced lemon (1 pc.) Sliced zucchini (2 pcs.) White wine (1 cup) Water (2 cups)

Salmon fillets (4 6-ounce pcs.) Kosher salt (1/4 tsp.)

Freshly ground pepper (1/4 tsp.)

Procedures:

1.   In a large Dutch oven, place the lemon, zucchini, onion, water and wine at the bottom of the oven.

2.   Season the salmon fillets with salt and pepper.

3.   In the meantime, fit a steamer rack over the vegetables in the oven and place it in medium to high heat until the liquid starts to boil.

4.   Reduce the heat from medium to low heat and carefully place the fillets in the rack. Cover the fillets and steam them for 8 – 10 minutes or until they are cooked through.

5.   Serve the fillets on top of the vegetables. Add poaching liquid and top it with sliced olives and garnish, if desired.

The steamed salmon fillets yield four servings. Each serving has 344 calories,

14.0   g fat, 121 mg cholesterol and 246 mg sodium.

Recipe # 2 – Sweet Potato and Black Bean Burgers with Lime Mayonnaise

Ingredients:

Low-fat or reduced-fat mayonnaise (1/2 cup) Lime (1 pc.)

Hot sauce (1/2 tsp.) Chopped small onion (1 pc.) Minced jalapeno (1 pc.) Ground cumin (2 tsp.) Minced garlic (2 tsp.)

Drained and mashed black beans (2 14.5 oz. cans) Raw sweet potato (2 cups)

Lightly beaten egg (1 pc.) Plain breadcrumbs (1 cup) Whole-wheat hamburger buns

Procedures:

1.   Set the oven rack 4 – 5 inches from the broiler then preheat the broiler at medium to high heat.

2.   Squeeze one lime into a mixing bowl and hot sauce and mayonnaise into the bowl. Stir the three ingredients well then refrigerate the mixture to set aside.

3.   Heat a large skillet in medium to high heat. Add the onion and cook for 3

– 4 minutes or until the onion is tender. Add the garlic, jalapeno and cumin then cook for 30 seconds.

4.   Add sweet potato, mashed beans, egg and ½ cup of breadcrumbs into a separate mixing bowl. Transfer the onion mixture from the skillet into the bowl and stir all ingredients well.

5.   Scoop the mixture and shape them into patties. Sprinkle the patties with the remaining breadcrumbs.

6.   Set patties on a lightly greased baking sheet and broil in the broiler for 8

-10 minutes. Turn over the patties then broil for another 8 – 10 minutes.

The patties should be cooked through and evenly browned.

7.   Place the patties on hamburger buns and add mayonnaise before serving.

The burgers can yield eight servings, with each burger having 344 calories, 8.4g fat, 28 mg cholesterol and 421 mg sodium.

Recipe # 3 – Red Pepper and Turkey Pasta

Ingredients:

Large red bell peppers (3 pcs.) Extra virgin olive oil (3 tbsp.) Chopped large onion (1 pc.) Minced garlic (2 tsp.) Chopped oregano (2 tbsp.) Red wine vinegar (1 tbsp.) Ground turkey (2 lbs.) Cooked rigatoni (2 lbs.)

Procedures:

1.   Cut bell pepper into halves, then remove the seeds and stem. Chop the peppers coarsely.

2.   Heat oil in a pan over medium heat from a large Dutch oven. Add the onion and peppers into the pan and cook for 20 minutes or until the peppers are very tender.

3.   Add garlic into the peppers and cook for five more minutes.

4.   Transfer the onion-and-pepper mixture into a blender and puree until smooth. Transfer the mixture back to the saucepan and reheat over low to medium heat.

5.   Add the vinegar and oregano. Stir well.

6.   Sauté ground turkey in a separate skillet with little oil and cook until the turkey begins to brown. Add the turkey into the red pepper sauce, mix it well and let it simmer for 20 minutes.

7.   Pour the pepper and turkey sauce over the cooked pasta then serve.

The red pepper and turkey pasta yields eight servings. Each serving has 629 calories, 15.1 g fat, 80 mg cholesterol, and 87 mg sodium.

Recipe # 4 – Weeknight Turkey Chili

Ingredients:

Chopped large onion (1 pc.) Minced garlic (1 tbsp.) Ground turkey (1 ½ cups) Water (2 cups)

Canned crushed tomatoes (1 28-oz. can) Drained kidney beans (1 16-oz. can) Chili powder (2 tbsp.)

Turmeric (2 tsp.)

Paprika (1 tsp.)

Oregano (1 tsp.) Ground cumin (1 tsp.) Hot sauce (1 tsp.)

Procedures:

1.   Cook onion in a large soup pot for 5 minutes, or until the onion starts to brown.

2.   Add garlic and cook for 30 seconds.

3.   Add ground turkey and stir continuously for 10 minutes until it is fully cooked.

4.   Add water and all the remaining ingredients into the soup pot and bring to a boil.

5.   Simmer with the pot uncovered for 30 – 45 minutes. Serve.

The turkey chili yields six servings. Each serving has 275 calories, 9.3 g fat, 80 mg cholesterol and 386 mg sodium.

Recipe # 5 – Brazil Nut-Crusted Tilapia with Sautéed Kale

Ingredients:

Roasted Brazil nuts (1/4 cup) Bread crumbs (1/2 cup)

Grated Parmesan cheese (2 tbsp.) Whole-grain mustard (1/4 cup) Tilapia fillets (1 ½ lbs.)

Sesame oil (1 tbsp.) Mashed garlic (1 clove) Chopped kale (1 ½ heads) Kosher salt (1/4 tsp.)

Toasted sesame seeds (2 tbsp.)

Procedures:

1.   Preheat oven to 400'F.

2.   Lightly grease a baking sheet. Set aside.

3.   Add Brazil nuts in a food processor and pulse the nuts until they are finely ground. Transfer the nuts into a mixing bowl and add parmesan cheese and breadcrumbs. Stir the ingredients well.

4.   Place tilapia fillets on the greased baking sheet and spread mustard on each fillet. Layer each fillet with the Brazil nut mixture.

5.   Bake the tilapia fillets for 8 – 10 minutes or until the fish is thoroughly cooked.

6.   In the meantime, heat a stainless-steel skillet over medium-high heat. Heat the sesame oil in the skillet for 15 seconds then add the garlic. Cook the garlic for 20 seconds then add kale. Stir the kale occasionally and cook for 7 -8 minutes.

7.   Add sesame seeds into the skillet and toss the mixture until the kale is fully combined with the seeds.

8.   Serve the fish fillets with a side of kale.

This meal yields six servings. Each serving has 255 calories, 11.2 g fat, 47 mg cholesterol and 400 mg sodium.

Recipe # 6 – Poached Eggs with Curried Vegetables

Ingredients:

Extra-virgin olive oil (2 tsp.) Chopped large onion (1 pc.) Minced garlic (1 clove) Yellow curry powder (1 tbsp.)

Sliced button mushrooms (1/2 lb.) Diced zucchini (2 medium pcs.) Drained chickpeas (1 14-oz. can) Water (1 cup)

White vinegar (1/2 tsp.) Large eggs (4 pcs.)

Crushed red pepper (1/8 tsp.)

Procedures:

1.   Sauté onion in a large non-stick skillet over medium to high heat for 4 -5 minutes, or until tender.

2.   Add garlic and cook for 30 seconds. Add the curry powder and stir it well with the garlic and onion. Cook for another 1- 2 minutes.

3.   Add mushrooms into the skillet and cook for another 5 minutes or until mushrooms become very tender.

4.   Add chickpeas, red pepper, zucchini and water into the skillet and bring the mixture into a boil. Then let it simmer for 15 – 20 minutes or until zucchini is very tender.

5.   In the meantime, add water in a separate saucepan to a depth of 3 inches. Boil the water, reduce heat, add vinegar and let it simmer.

6.   Crack the eggs and slide each egg into the water one at a time, making sure it touches the surface of the water. Simmer the eggs for 3 -5 minutes, then remove the eggs with a large spoon.

7.   Serve the eggs with a side of vegetables.

This meal yields four servings. Each serving has 261 calories, 9.1 g fat, 185 mg cholesterol and 373 mg sodium.

Recipe # 7 - Quinoa & Turkey Stuffed Peppers

Serves 6; Preparation time – 55 minutes

Ingredients:

Uncooked quinoa (1 cup) Water (2 cups)

Salt (½ tsp)

Fully-cooked, diced smoked turkey sausage (½ pound) Chicken stock (½ cup)

Extra-virgin olive oil (¼ cup) Chopped pecans, toasted (3 tbsp) Chopped fresh parsley (2 tbsp) Chopped fresh rosemary (2 tsp) Red bell peppers (3 pcs)

Procedures:

1.   Using a large saucepan, stir the quinoa, salt, and water together. Boil the mixture in high-heat. Once boiling, reduce the heat and cover the saucepan. Simmer for about 15 minutes or until the water is almost completely absorbed.

2.   Remove the cover and let the dish stand for 5 more minutes. Stir in the sausage together with the rest of the ingredients.

3.   Fill the pepper with cooked quinoa mixture and put it on a slightly greased 13 x 9" baking dish. Bake the stuffed peppers for 15 minutes at 3500F heat.

Recipe # 8 - Poached Black Sesame Salmon and Bok Choy Broth

Serves 2

Ingredients:

Wild salmon (2 quarter pound pcs) Seafood stock (3 cups)

Lime, thinly sliced (1 pc)

Whole black peppercorns (10 pcs) Bok choy (2 heads)

Lime juice (from 1 pc of lime) Salt and pepper, to taste

Toasted black sesame seeds, for garnishing

Preparation:

1.   In a heavy pot or deep skillet, mix the lime, peppercorn and seafood stock. Bring to a boil over high heat. Once boiling, lower the heat to a simmer immediately. Cover the pot and cook for another 5 minutes.

2.   Season the salmon with salt & pepper, and then gently lower it to a simmering liquid. Be sure that the filets are ¾ covered (at the very least). Lower the heat to an even gentler simmer. Then cover the pot and cook for another 6 more minutes or until the salmon is opaque all over (or when you are able to flake it using a fork). Take the salmon out of the liquid. Prepare a towel-lined plate and set the salmon on top.

3.   Turn up the heat to medium setting to make the broth simmer at a steady pace. Toss in the bok choy heads and let them cook for around 3 minutes or until soft (not mushy so it would still result to a good bite). Remove the bok choy from the simmering liquid.

4.   Turn up the heat once more, this time to medium high setting and continue cooking the broth for another 3 minutes. Put the lime juice in, then turn the heat off.

5.   Halve the salmon and bok choy into two shallow bowls. Using a ladle, pour ¼ to ½ cup of broth on each bowl. Finish off by garnishing with black sesame seeds. Serve hot.

Recipe # 9 – Almond Chicken

Serves 1; Preparation time – 30 minutes

Boneless chicken breast, sliced (3 oz.) Broccoli flowerets, steamed (2 cups) Olive oil (1 1/2 tsp)

Green bell pepper, chopped (1 pc) Red bell pepper, chopped (1 pc) Onion, chopped (3/4 cup)

Garlic, minced (1 clove)

Cherry tomatoes, halved (1 cup) Salt & pepper, to taste

Sliced almonds (2 tsp)

Procedures:

1.	Steam the broccoli. At the same time, heat some olive oil in a saute pan.

2.	Put the chicken, red and green pepper, garlic and onion in the pan and saute until the chicken is cooked inside and out, and the veggies are cooked al dente.

3.	Toss in the steamed broccoli and tomatoes. Top with almonds.

Recipe # 10 – Rice Pilaf

Serves 3

Ingredients:

Olive oil (1 tsp)

Finely chopped onion (2 tbsp.) Chicken broth (1 cup)

Zone orzo (1/2 cup) Dried thyme (1/4 tsp) Salt & pepper to taste

Procedures:

1.   Get a small saucepan and heat oil under medium heat setting. Add finely chopped onions. Cook until tender, stirring frequently.

2.   Put a tablespoon of broth or as necessary.

3.   Boil a cup of broth, then add Zone orzo. Stir until the broth is almost completely absorbed. That should take around 5 minutes.

4.   Toss in the sautéed onion, salt & pepper, and thyme. Reduce heat and continue cooking until the broth is completely absorbed.

5.   Gently fluff the rice with fork gently before serving.

Recipe # 11 – Beef Barbecue w/ Onions

Serves 1; Preparation time – 45 minutes

Ingredients:

Olive oil, divided (1 1/2 tsp) Beef, eye of round (3 oz.) Tomato puree (1/2 cup) Worcestershire sauce (1 tsp) Cider vinegar (1/3 tsp)

Chili powder (1/3 tsp) Cumin (1/8 tsp) Oregano (1/8 tsp)

Onion, in half rings (1 cup) Garlic, minced (1 clove) Mushrooms (1 cup)

Unsalted vegetable stock (2 tsp) White wine vinegar (2 tsp) Snow peas (1 cup)

Procedures:

1.   Heat ½ tsp of oil in a skillet, then place the beef. Cook the beef until it is no longer pink

1.   Add the Worcestershire sauce, puree, chili powder, cider vinegar, oregano, and cumin into the skillet.

2.   Cover and allow to simmer for about 5 minutes or just until the sauce forms.

3.   Get another skillet and put the remaining oil, garlic, and onion. Cook until the onion becomes tender.

4.   Add garlic, onion, beef stock, white wine vinegar, and mushrooms to the beef. Cover the dish and allow to cook for about 8 more minutes. Midway or after around 5 minutes, add the snow peas. Occasionally stir to blend the flavors well.

Recipe # 12 - Citrus Tofu Salad

Serves 1; Preparation time – 25 minutes

Olive oil, divided (1 tsp) Worcestershire sauce (1/2 tsp) Celery salt (1/8 tsp)

Extra firm tofu, ½" (6 oz.) Asparagus spears – 1" (1 1/2 cups) Celery, sliced (1 1/2 cups)

Garlic, minced (1/2 tsp)

Hot pepper sauce, dash (1/2 tsp) Paprika (1/2 tsp)

Lemon herb seasoning (1/8 tsp) Dried dill (1/2 tsp)

Salt & pepper, to taste Romaine lettuce (5 cups)

Mandarin orange segments, in water (1/3 cup)

Procedures:

1.   Get a medium-sized saute pan and spray with olive oil. Then, heat ½ tsp oil.

2.   Blend the Worcestershire sauce, tofu, and celery salt in. Stir fry until all sides are crusted and browned.

3.   Get another non-stick saute pan and heat the remaining oil. Stir fry the celery, asparagus, garlic, paprika, hot pepper sauce, dill, salt & pepper, and lemon herb seasoning until the veggies are crisp and tender.

4.   Put some lettuce on a serving plate, with the orange segments evenly distributed over it.

5.   To finish, top first with some veggie mixture, then finally with tofu.

6.   Serve and enjoy!

Recipe # 13 – American Chop Suey w/ Salad

Serves 1; Preparation time – 20 minutes

Ingredients:

Zone fusilli (2/3 cup) Olive oil (1 tsp)

Celery, chopped (1/2 stalk) Onion, diced (3 tbsp.) Garlic, minced (1 clove)

Red bell pepper, diced (3 tbsp.)

Extra-lean turkey breast, ground (1 1/2 oz.) Cooking spray

Canned tomatoes, diced (1/2 - 14.5 oz. can) Crushed red pepper flakes (1/4 tsp)

Fresh chopped basil (1/4 tsp) Salt & pepper, to taste

Freshly-squeezed lemon juice (1 tbsp.) Extra virgin olive oil (1 tsp)

Lettuce (1/2 cup) Tomato (1/4 pc) Cucumber (1/4 pc)

Procedures:

1.   Cook the Zone fusilli for 3 to 4 minutes. Set aside after draining.

2.   Heat oil in a skillet under medium-high temperature setting. Toss in the onion and celery. Allow to cook for a few minutes before adding the peppers and garlic.

3.   Remove the vegetables from the pan. Using a cooking spray, drizzle and saute the turkey until its color is no longer pinkish. Bring the vegetable mix back into the pan together with the partially cooked fusilli.

4.   Top with crushed red pepper and canned tomatoes. Stir everything well before covering and allowing to simmer for another 8 minutes.

5.   Top the dish with fresh basil right before serving, preferably with a small salad side.

Recipe # 14 – Antipasto Salad

Serves 3; Preparation time – 20 minutes

Ingredients:

Iceberg lettuce, shredded (1 1/2 heads) Celery, sliced (2 cups)

Carrots, sliced thin (3/4 cup) Mushrooms, sliced (3 cups) Onions, in half rings (1 cup)

Red bell peppers, in half rings (2 1/4 cups) Garbanzo beans, canned (3/4 cup)

Light tuna chunks, in water (2 oz.)

Low-fat mozzarella cheese – shredded (2 oz.) Sliced turkey (3 oz.)

Extra-lean ham slice (2 oz.)

Dried basil - crushed in palm of hand (2 tsp) Extra virgin olive oil, drizzle (3 tsp)

No-Fat Tasty Dressing - (1/4 cup)

Procedures:

1.   Get 3 large-sized oval plates and set a lettuce bed on each one. Put the carrots, celery, mushrooms, red pepper, onions, and garbanzo beans on the bed of lettuce, forming a vertical line starting from the right side going to the left side of the plate.

2.   Next, put the cheese, tuna, ham, and turkey on the plates, distributed evenly, using the strips of red bell pepper as divider.

3.   Using your palm, crush the basil to release its freshness, and then sprinkle over the plates. Sprinkle a tsp of olive oil on all the plates. Whisk the dressing quickly before pouring on the salad.

Recipe # 15 – Asian Stir Fried Chicken

Serves 2; Preparation time – 30 minutes

Ingredients:

Broccoli, chopped (3 cups) Olive oil (2 tsp)

Skinless, boneless chicken breast (cut to bite sized pieces (7 oz.) Garlic, pressed (2 cloves)

Water chestnuts, sliced (3/4 cup) Mushrooms, sliced (8 oz.)

Red bell pepper, sliced (1 pc) Snow peas (1 cup)

Scallions, sliced (1/2 cup) Low sodium soy sauce (2 tsp)

Mandarin orange sections (1/2 cup) Toasted sesame oil (1 tsp)

Procedures:

1.   Steam the broccoli for about 3 to 4 minutes. To stop cooking, rinse with some cold water. Set the broccoli aside and allow it to drain in a strainer.

2.   Get a large-sized skillet and heat some olive oil under medium heat setting.

3.   Add the garlic and chicken, and allow to cook until the juices are running clear. Then, add mushrooms, water chestnuts, scallions, snow peas, soy sauce, and pepper into the mix. Continue to cook until the veggies are tender. If necessary, add some vegetable stock in 1 tsp increments. Stir the sections of Mandarin orange in, together with the toasted sesame oil.

4.   Transfer to a large plate and serve.

Conclusion

A person undergoing an anti-inflammatory diet has to eat healthy meals that follow his dietician's prescription. However, these meals should also be tasty and palatable enough for the dieter to enjoy. With this recipe book, you have a hundred percent assurance that you will enjoy healthy and delicious meals.

I hope this book was able to help you to feed patients who suffer from rheumatoid arthritis and other serious conditions. I also hope the recipes are easy and comprehensible enough for culinary beginners to follow.

The next step is to customize the meals and try out other ingredients that you or your patient may prefer. However, it is best to check if you have allergic reactions to certain food or ingredients. It is also best to consult a dietician before serving customized meals.

Finally, if you enjoyed this book, please take the time to share your thoughts and post a positive review on Amazon. It'd be greatly appreciated!

Thank you and good luck!

CPSIA information can be obtained
at www.ICGtesting.com
Printed in the USA
BVHW090221260621
610448BV00006B/1535